N259·5·£12.00

KT-486-038

0108933

Nurse
Manager

A Practical Guide to Better Employee Relations

Books are to be returned on or before
the last date below.

June Blankenship Pugh, MS, RN, CS

Nursing Resources Coordinator
Veterans Administration Medical Center
Nashville, Tennessee

Mary Ann Woodward-Smith, MSN, RN, CS

Mental Health Clinic Coordinator
Veterans Administration Medical Center
Nashville, Tennessee

1989
W. B. SAUNDERS COMPANY
Harcourt Brace Jovanovich, Inc.
Philadelphia • London • Toronto • Montreal • Sydney

HAROLD BRIDGES LIBRARY
S. MARTIN'S COLLEGE
LANCASTER

072162863X

W. B. SAUNDERS COMPANY
Harcourt Brace Jovanovich, Inc.

The Curtis Center
Independence Square West
Philadelphia, PA 19106

Editor: Thomas Eoyang
Designer: William Boehm
Production Manager: Carolyn Naylor
Manuscript Editor: Sarah Fitz-Hugh
Cover Artist: Brett MacNaughton

Nurse Manager:
A Practical Guide to Better Employee Relations   ISBN 0-7216-2863-X
© 1989 by W. B. Saunders Company. Copyright by W. B. Saunders Company. Copyright under the Uniform Copyright Convention. Simultaneously published in Canada. All rights reserved. This book is protected by copyright. No part of it may be reproduced, stored in a retrieval system, or transmitted in any form or by any means, electronic, mechanical, photocopying, recording, or otherwise, without written permission from the publisher. Made in the United States of America.

Last digit is the print number: 9   8   7   6   5   4   3   2   1

Dedication

*To the nurse managers
at the Nashville Veterans Administration Medical Center,
who gave us opportunities to try our ideas
and taught us as much as we taught them.*

Acknowledgments

Goals are more easily accomplished with the support of others. For this reason we are grateful to our husbands, Jim and Gary, our typist, Marylou Kintner, and our editor, Thomas Eoyang.

Foreword
A Vision of the Future

Health care has become enormously complex, especially with the implementation of the prospective payment system. Adding to this complexity is health care's lack of awareness of itself as a service in the sense that a service is, in part, intangible and people-intensive. The value of the service is influenced, in part, by "value-added" interactions among patients and health-care personnel.

With hospitals and other health-care agencies becoming more service oriented, health care becoming more sophisticated, and the nursing shortage becoming more complex, nursing must emphasize better employee relations and "managing the environment." Nurse managers at every level are in crucial front-line positions.

There is a need for practical, readable texts targeted for nurse managers, who come to their positions with a variety of educational backgrounds. Nurse managers must help nurses feel good about themselves and their work, through clearly stated mutual goals and open, honest, timely feedback. This book gives step-by-step instructions on how to instill these feelings.

Front-line nurse managers serve as role models and greatly influence the environments of their units. Therefore, their use of cognitive restructuring and assertive communication techniques as discussed in this book can create an environment where stress can be reduced and employee and patient satisfaction enhanced.

Nurse managers need to become more sensitive to the differences and inherent conflicts between their managerial roles and their clinical roles. This book stresses the need for nurse managers to avoid "taking care of" employees, to create support systems through networking, and to establish power bases within the workplace.

Nurse managers who utilize the skills presented in this book will create exciting, stimulating work environments in which employees will feel good about themselves and will have opportunities for professional growth.

COLLEEN CONWAY-WELCH, PhD, FAAN
Professor and Dean
Vanderbilt University School of Nursing
Nashville, Tennessee

Introduction
A Guide to Better
Employee Relations

Nursing is a people-oriented discipline. It is through people that nursing achieves its purpose. This is especially true for nurse managers who must work with and through a number of people and many disciplines in the hospital setting to assure the best possible care to patients, support for their families, leadership for the nursing staff, and collaboration with other health care personnel.

In their work with nurse managers at a major tertiary care Veterans Administration Medical Center, the authors over time have provided guidance and useful information to assist nurse managers in their work. These two teachers have given much and have gained much in the process. Because of this dynamic exchange and a positive collective experience, this guide is shared with you in the hope that it will enable many others to achieve maximum outcomes as they work successfully with people.

This book is timely, for in today's health care system, and in the foreseeable future, competition for nursing personnel is keen. Those settings that emphasize and act on improving employee relations are preferred. When nurses relate to other nurses in a wholesome manner, good results accrue as they care for others. Many thoughts on how to achieve better employee relations are offered.

VERNICE FERGUSON, RN, MA, FAAN, FRCN
Deputy Assistant Chief Medical Director
for Nursing Programs
The Veterans Administration
Washington, DC

Preface
How This Book Can Help You

"I was taught how to deal with problem patients in nursing school, but I wasn't taught how to deal with problem employees." "I've got patients to take care of. I don't have time to deal with employee problems." Statements like these are echoed by nurses in management positions across the country. In a sense, all nurses are managers.

The primary focus in nursing schools, however, is the management of patient care. Little emphasis is placed on the management of employees. Whether you are a charge nurse, head nurse, or director of nursing, you have earned your position by demonstrating your excellent patient skills. But chances are you have learned to be a manager through on-the-job training. The goal of this book is to present skills that will improve your ability to relate well with your employees. Upon completion you will know:

1. How an assertive nurse manager looks, thinks, feels, and acts.
2. The difference between assertive, aggressive, and passive managerial styles.

3. Assertive verbal and nonverbal communication techniques.
4. How to use positive, rational self-talk to reduce stress and to solve personnel problems.
5. How to motivate your employees.
6. How to set effective goals through mutual participation by you and your employees.
7. How to give your employees positive and negative feedback in order to improve performance.
8. How to avoid falling into the trap of "nursing" your employees.
9. How to develop a supportive network for yourself and your staff.
10. How to develop and utilize a power base to benefit you, your organization, and your employees.

We have some basic beliefs that are the foundation upon which this book is written.

1. Assertive communication is the most effective method of communicating with employees.
2. Assertive communication is a learned behavior or skill.
3. Learning a new behavior is anxiety producing and involves taking risks.
4. All of us are responsible for our own behavior and the consequences of that behavior.
5. No one can accept responsibility for another person's behavior.
6. In making a decision, you must determine whether the potential results are worth the perceived risks and accept responsibility for that decision.
7. Our reactions to people and events are directly related to the messages we give ourselves about these events.
8. People perform better and are more motivated on their jobs when they know what is expected of them and are given both positive and negative feedback regarding performance.

9. Developing a supportive network and utilizing power are important skills for today's nurse manager.

If these premises are valid for you, this book will prove to be a valuable addition to your library. We suggest that you read it through and then reread each section, practicing the skills as they are presented. Keep the book handy for those days when your managerial momentum needs a boost.

> We're reminded of the story about a man who is being chased by a tiger. As he comes to a steep cliff, the tiger is hot on his heels. His choices are to either jump or be eaten by the tiger. He jumps, but luckily there's a twig sticking out of the cliff and he manages to grab it. The tiger is leaning over the cliff, trying to get him. He can feel the tiger's hot breath on his neck, and he can see the jagged rocks below. Naturally the man resorts to prayer. He says, "Lord, if you'll just get me out of this situation, I'll do anything you say." Out of the blue comes a booming voice commanding, "Let go of the branch!" The man studies the jagged rocks again, looks up, and asks, "Is there anyone else up there?"

You must be willing to let go of the branches of old behavior or ideas if you are to develop the skills required to be an effective nurse manager. You've been asking for help with your employee relations. Are you ready? Let go of the branch!

JUNE BLANKENSHIP PUGH
MARY ANN WOODWARD-SMITH

Authors' note: We have chosen to use the pronoun "she" throughout the book since the majority of nurses are women.

Prologue

. . . Once upon a time in a large urban medical center, a group of head nurses, supervisors, and nursing administrators got together for the purpose of developing a concise yet comprehensive list of skills that would serve as a guide to better nurse manager–employee relations. When they were finished, the nurses were proud of their work. "This is a very good list," said one of the head nurses. "I wish more nurse managers could see it." "Yes," agreed the director of nursing. "If all nurse managers applied these skills, they would greatly benefit themselves, their employees, and their organizations." The in-service director said enthusiastically, "Someone should write a book about these skills!"

And so someone did . . .

Contents

Foreword   A Vision of the Future. vii

Introduction   A Guide to Better Employee
Relations ix

Preface   How This Book Can Help You xi

Prologue   Once upon a Time. xv

PART I   THE ESSENTIAL SKILLS

1   Passive, Aggressive or Assertive
Nurse Manager: *It's a Matter of Style* . . . 3

2   Assertive Verbal Skills: *Do You Say
What You Mean?* 13

3   Nonverbal Communication: *Does
Your Behavior Speak So Loudly,
They Can't Hear What You Say?* 20

4   Managerial Listening Response:
             Two Ears and One Mouth 25

5   Rational Thinking: *Management
             Can Be Fun — I Think* 30

6   Stress Management: *Curing the
             Super-Nurse Syndrome* 35

7   Motivation: *Creating a Team* 42

8   Goal Setting: *If You Don't Know
             Where You Are Going, How Will You
             Know When You Get There?* 51

9   Feedback: *Staying On Course*. 62

PART II   PUTTING IT ALL TOGETHER

10   Clinical Skills Versus Management
             Skills: *With Everything Else You
             Have to Do, Why Would You Adopt a
             Monkey?* 73

11   Networking: *What Counts Is Not
             What You Know, But Who You Know
             Who Knows What You Need to Know* . . 80

12   Power: *It All Adds Up* 86

Bibliography   92

Index   95

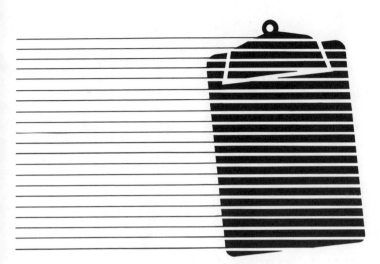

Part 1

The Essential Skills

1

Passive, Aggressive, or Assertive Nurse Manager
It's a matter of style

lthough there are other styles of management, we believe that assertive management offers the best way to feel good about yourself as a manager and the best way to help your employees feel good about themselves and their jobs. To understand the functioning of the assertive nurse manager, we will begin with a definition:

An assertive nurse manager supervises employees by stating expectations and giving positive and negative feedback regarding performance. She communicates openly, honestly, and directly, without violating the employees' rights to benefit the organization and to reach their full potential.

To better understand this definition, let's look at each component.

Stating expectations	Set goals with employees.
Positive and negative feedback	After goals have been set, let your employees know how they are doing in relation to meeting those goals.
Regarding performance	Give feedback that's always performance related and that avoids personality issues.
Without violating the employees' rights to benefit the organization	Employees have the right to do their jobs. When people are hired, they begin with the intention of doing a good job. A manager can either facilitate or interfere with employees' functioning. Setting goals and giving feedback in an open, honest, and direct fashion will enhance an employee's ability to benefit the organization.
To reach their full potential	By managing assertively you will increase your employees' self-esteem and job satisfaction, thereby helping them to become all they can be.

Management Styles

The best way to understand an assertive management style is to compare and contrast it with passive and aggressive management styles. While none of us is always passive, aggressive, or even assertive, you have a pattern of communicating with employees that best defines your management style.

Assertive Style

The assertive nurse manager places a high priority on producing results but also devotes time and attention to the people needed to produce those results. Her goal is communicating without violating her rights or the rights of others. Consequently she earns the respect of both her supervisors and her employees.

Aggressive Style

The aggressive manager is guided by a different goal. Her aim is to get what she and the organization want. Her priorities are clearly focused on results. For this reason she may be looked upon with favor by her organization —until unhappy, disgruntled employees begin to request transfers. Since employees' needs are not a high priority, she does little to help them reach their full potential. Management by intimidation will never earn popularity or respect.

Contrasting Management Styles			
	Passive Nurse Manager	**Aggressive Nurse Manager**	**Assertive Nurse Manager**
Goal	No conflict	To get what I want	Communication without violation
Action Priorities	To meet the needs of the employees	To meet the needs of the organization	To meet the needs of the organization and employees
Short-Term Consequences	Nurse manager loses and employees win	Nurse manager wins and employees lose	Nurse manager and employees win
Long-Range Consequences	Nurse manager and employees lose because of increased stress and decreased job satisfaction	Nurse manager and employees lose because of increased stress and decreased job satisfaction	Nurse manager and employees continue to win because of decreased stress and increased job satisfaction
Interpersonal Relationships	May be well liked but is not respected	Is not liked or respected	May be well liked but is definitely well respected

Passive Style

A passive nurse manager aims for the goal of no conflict. Because she desires peace at any price, she places priority on what the employees want, often at the expense of producing good results. While the organization may be displeased with her inefficiency, her employees will enjoy her laid-back attitude. Eventually even she will discover that she cannot always ensure everyone's satisfaction and happiness. Because she never clearly communicates expectations or gives performance-related feedback, her employees do not have the opportunity to reach their full potential. In her efforts to be well liked, she will never be well respected.

Examples Contrasting Management Styles

If you think of the nurse manager's response as the remedy for a managerial problem, you would want to choose a response that has the most immediate desired results with the least number of side effects. On this basis, evaluate the effectiveness of each nurse manager in the following three examples.

Situation

At 11:45 A.M. Dr. Jones calls the head nurse complaining that his diabetic patient, Mr. Smith, has not received foot care since admission two days ago. Dr. Jones is very angry. He demands that this oversight be taken care of before he makes rounds again at 3:00 P.M. The nursing assistant assigned to Mr. Smith is scheduled for lunch at noon. He's a union steward.

Responses

Passive (no-conflict) Nurse Manager

The head nurse is visibly upset by the phone call. Dr. Jones is certainly not someone she wants to cross. She dreads confronting the nursing assistant, who is always reminding her of his "legal rights."

Head Nurse: Excuse me, Fred.

Nursing Assistant: (hurriedly) I know, it's time for me to go to lunch.

Head Nurse: Well, yes, but, uh, Dr. Jones called. Well, uh, I know you've been busy, but have you had a chance to do Mr. Smith's foot care?

Nursing Assistant: Nope! See you later. By the way, I'll be late getting back today. We've got a steward's meeting at 12:30.

Head Nurse: Well, uh, okay, I guess. (Walks away talking to herself) I guess I'll do that foot care myself. It might be better for me to do it, anyway. I want to make sure it's done right.

In this example, the head nurse achieved her goal. She avoided conflict and made the doctor happy. If you examine the long-range consequences, however, you will find that the head nurse may have to deal with unpleasant side effects that were not a part of her goal. This head nurse is paying a high price to avoid conflict. Chances are she feels resentful because no one appreciates her efforts to keep everyone happy. Because she tries to handle too much herself, she is overworked. She labors under a great deal of self-imposed stress, which will eventually take its toll on her physically if she does not leave the job first.

Aggressive (get-what-I-want) Nurse Manager

The head nurse is angered by the phone call. She sets high standards, likes to keep the doctors happy, and views this report as an attack on her competency. She sees the nursing assistant headed for lunch. She approaches him with obvious anger.

Head Nurse: Where do you think you are going? I've been getting complaints about you all morning.

Nursing Assistant: (defensively) Who?

Head Nurse: Never mind! Go do Mr. Smith's foot care! Now!

Nursing Assistant: (angrily) It's my lunch break and I've got a steward's meeting at 12:30.

Head Nurse: Patient care comes first around here. I want that foot care done before you go anywhere!

Nursing Assistant: (stomps away talking to self) I'll bet that patient's been complaining about me!

Head Nurse: (to herself) You have to be tough with these people. Dr. Jones will be pleased.

This head nurse got what she and the doctor wanted—results. The head nurse in this example is building resistance among her staff. Although she is interested in results, it will become harder and harder to produce the results she desires without the cooperation of her staff. When she pushes as hard as she can and uses all of her "big guns" to get the job done, what methods will be left for her to try? The stress of her job must also weigh heavily on her shoulders because, in a sense, she is carrying it all alone.

Assertive (communication-without-violation) Nurse Manager

The head nurse checks the schedule and the patient to verify the information. She is annoyed that her colleague, Dr. Jones, has been put in this position. She is puzzled by the nursing assistant's poor performance.

Head Nurse: I see you're about to leave for lunch. I need to talk with you first.

Nursing Assistant: I'm in a hurry. Remember, I told you about that steward's meeting at 12:30?

Head Nurse: Yes, I remember. Dr. Jones just called. He was very upset because Mr. Smith has not received foot care since admission. I checked the patient myself and I found Dr. Jones's report to be accurate. Looking at the assignment sheet, I see that Mr. Smith has been your patient since admission. Let me tell you how I feel. First, I feel angry because Mr. Smith's foot care was not done, and we both know how important foot care is for a diabetic. Second, I feel angry because I don't like having a colleague call me and report that a patient has not received proper nursing care. (Pause) Now let me tell you something else: You are much better than this (touches employee's arm). You usually pay close attention to these special treatments. Mr. Smith's foot care must be done before Dr. Jones makes rounds at 3 o'clock. You haven't had lunch and you have a meeting at 12:30. What do you suggest?*

Nursing Assistant: I feel bad about this. I'll do the foot care now. I can take my lunch to the meeting.

---

*Adapted from Blanchard K, Johnson S. "One Minute Reprimand." *In The One Minute Manager*. New York, Berkley Books, 1986.

> *Head Nurse*: **Great. I won't give it another thought. I know I can depend on you.**

This head nurse met all the goals identified in the definition of the assertive nurse manager. She was open, honest, and direct in her communication of negative feedback and expectations. She facilitated the employee's right to benefit the organization, and she allowed the employee to participate in resolving the problem. It is no accident that she has a spirit of teamwork and cooperation on her ward. Her employees feel her concern for them, and they all work together to produce good results. This head nurse experiences a lesser degree of stress and a greater degree of job satisfaction.

These examples illustrate that the assertive managerial response is the one most likely to have the desired results with the least undesirable long-range consequences. Being assertive will not guarantee success, but it will build your confidence and improve your odds for success.

Making Assertiveness Your Management Style

Assertiveness is a skill—a learned behavior, not a talent. None of us was born knowing how to be assertive. Having a knowledge of assertiveness is essential, but not enough. This book gives you the principles of being an assertive nurse manager. Developing the skill will be up to you.

If assertiveness is a new skill for you, you may want to

create a peer support network where you can role-play assertiveness techniques. You can also start practicing assertiveness in everyday occurrences with your employees. Start with simple situations in which the outcome is not of crucial importance. Gradually work your way up to more complicated, critical situations. Just as with any skill, the more you practice, the more adept you will become at being an assertive nurse manager.

2

Assertive Verbal Skills
Do you say what you mean?

There were two bachelor brothers, John and Joe, who lived in the country with their mother and old cat. Now John and Joe never ventured out very much, but one day John decided he would go on vacation. John had never been away from home before, and the whole family's anxiety was high, but he promised he would call home every night and check on everyone.

The first night he called home and talked with brother Joe. "Joe, how's Mama?" "Oh, she's fine, John." "Good. How's the cat?" "Well, John, I have terrible news. Mama and the cat went out on the road to get the mail, and a car came flying down the road, hit the cat, and killed him."

John was naturally stunned. When he had recovered somewhat, he reprimanded his brother sternly: "Joe, that's no way to tell me bad news. You know how I loved that cat. You should have broken it to me gently. Tonight when I called home you could have said, 'Brother, the cat is on the roof, and we can't get him down.' The next night you could have said, 'Well, the cat fell off the roof, and we had to take him to the vet.' Then the third night you could have said, 'I'm sorry, John, the vet did all he could, but the cat died.' You see, that way you would be breaking the bad news to me gently." Joe apologized, "Well, okay, John. I'm sorry. I'll try to do better." The next night when John called home he asked cheerfully, "Hi, Joe, how's Mama?" Joe paused a minute. "Well, John, Mama's on the roof."

We tell this story to illustrate the point that the words you choose are important. As a manager you are in a position of authority and your position makes it even more critical to carefully consider your verbal communication. Some of the more difficult areas in employee communication are giving feedback, denying a request, dealing with criticism, and negotiating a compromise. You can learn some specific assertive verbal skills that will help you improve your communication in these areas.*

I-Messages versus You-Messages

Your employees will be more receptive to your feedback when you phrase it as an *I-message*. I-messages take responsibility for your own reactions, feelings, and needs (I think, I feel, I want). *You-messages* imply blame and accusation (You said, You did, You should not have).

---

*The skills discussed are adapted from Smith M. *When I Say No I Feel Guilty.* New York, Bantam Books, 1975.

Practice turning you-messages into I-messages. Instead of saying to a staff nurse, "You never get to work on time," you could say, "I'm concerned that you are frequently late." Instead of telling a nursing assistant, "You know you cannot go to lunch until all the patients are fed," you could say, "I do not like for you to go to lunch before all the patients are fed." Instead of saying to a doctor, "How do you expect anyone to read these orders? You're going to cause a nurse to make a big medication error one of these days!", you could say, "Please write your orders more legibly. I'm concerned that a nurse may make a medication error." Remember I-messages take responsibility for your feelings, whereas you-messages cast blame on others.

Firm Persistence

As a manager there will be times when your employees will make requests that you will have to deny. Some managers find it difficult to say no, especially nurse managers, since nurses in their role as caretakers tend to be concerned about pleasing people. A technique that can be very useful in learning to say no is *firm persistence*. Calmly repeat over and over again what you want or what your position is until the other person agrees or gives up, or until you reach a compromise. You should maintain a low-level relaxed voice when using firm persistence. You do not want to get into a shouting match.

Let's suppose you have an employee who wants the weekend off and you have to deny her request. The dialogue using firm persistence might go as follows:

Staff Nurse: **I really need to be off this weekend. I just** found out my family is coming from out of town, and I haven't seen them in three years.

Head Nurse: I can understand your feelings, but I can't give you this weekend off. What other options do you have?

Staff Nurse: I just have to be off. They won't understand me working after they drove 1,000 miles to see me.

Head Nurse: It sounds like a difficult situation, but I can't give you this weekend off. What other options do you have?

Staff Nurse: Why can't you? I never ask to be off on weekends. I'm always willing to work and let other people have the weekends off.

Head Nurse: I appreciate your willingness to work in the past, but I can't give you this weekend off. Have you thought of any other options?

Staff Nurse: Please, I thought we were friends. I've done favors for you before.

Head Nurse: I can certainly understand your disappointment, but I can't give you this weekend off. I'm willing to discuss other options.

It is important to remember that it is not always necessary to respond to an employee's questions or comments. You simply maintain your position. What are the benefits of firm persistence? It puts you in control of the situation and keeps you from being manipulated. You do not have to spend time rehearsing arguments beforehand in order to be ready to deal with a conflictual situation. As with all assertive skills, you will need to practice firm persistence for it to become a technique you can use comfortably.

Dealing with Criticism

As a nurse manager there may be days when you feel that everyone is out to get you. Criticism is coming from all directions—doctors, your staff, administrators, patients, families, and visitors. The typical response to criticism is increased anxiety and defensiveness. Here are assertive techniques that will help you avoid becoming anxious and defensive when being criticized:

Agreeing with the Possibility

Calmly acknowledge to your critic that there possibly is some truth in what he or she is saying. However, you remain the judge of your own behavior.

> *Staff Nurse*: **I don't think the time schedule is fair.**
> *Head Nurse*: **Possibly it could be more fair.**

Asking for More Information

You acknowledge the criticism and clarify by asking for more information. What, when, where, and/or how?

> *Staff Nurse*: **I think you showed partiality in the time schedule.**
> *Head Nurse*: **I'm sure I could have done a better job. What specifically did you notice?**

Owning the Mistake

You simply accept and acknowledge your own faults and mistakes.

> *Staff Nurse*: **Sue has had four weekends off in the past two months and I've only had one.**
> *Head Nurse*: **You're right. I made a mistake. I'll look at the schedule and get back to you tomorrow.**

These techniques prevent situations from escalating, help you deal with manipulative criticism, and gain more from constructive criticism. Because the techniques decrease your anxiety and defensiveness, you become an approachable manager who is open and receptive to suggestions from employees.

Compromise Through Assertive Negotiation

As a manager, the ability to reach a *compromise through assertive negotiation* is an essential skill. The best compromise is one in which all parties involved feel that they have, at the most, gotten all or some part of what they wanted. But at the very least, they feel that their ideas, opinions, and feelings have been listened to and respected.

Example

Staff Nurse: I would like two weeks off in June. I want to spend some time with my children while they're out of school.

Head Nurse: I can understand your desire to be off with your children this summer. I will be glad to give you some time off, but I can't give you two full weeks in June. I could give you a week in June and a week in July or August.

Staff Nurse: Okay. I'd like a week in June and a week in August.

All compromises will not be as straightforward as this example. Each of us holds certain ethical and moral values that are very important to us. You should never compromise if your self-worth or self-respect will be diminished.

3

Nonverbal Communication

Does your behavior speak so loudly, they can't hear what you say?

You often choose your words carefully in an attempt to elicit a favorable response, to be taken seriously, or to be understood correctly. You probably pay less attention to your nonverbal communication. However, behavioral scientists tell us that the majority of our communications are nonverbal. Thus your employees respond mostly to your nonverbal language. Your carefully chosen words may be drowned out by the roar of your nonverbal behavior, which is largely out of your awareness. You can, however, develop nonverbal communication skills so that your body language becomes consistent with your words and actually reinforces the verbal message you are sending.

Behavior Cues

Although your words may be assertive, if your behavior gives a different message, then your listener will most likely respond to the behavior cues, and your verbal message will be ineffective. Here are some of the behavior cues that you should be aware of.

- Tone of Voice; Is it timid, demanding, or confident?
- Eye Contact; Is it avoidant, staring and intimidating, or comfortably direct?
- Gestures; Are they nervous, threatening, or used for emphasis?
- Posture; Is it meek and humble, rigid and tense, or comfortably erect and confident?
- Distance; Is it exaggerated and barricaded, crowding and intimidating, or appropriate and considerate?

For a dramatic illustration of the impact of nonverbal behaviors, make the following statement three times, changing only the nonverbal behavior to make the message passive, aggressive, or assertive. You can practice the statement in front of a mirror or with a friend.

Statement

I am your new head nurse. I'm going to be meeting with each of you to set some mutual goals, so be working on some individual goals before our meeting. I will also be giving you frequent feedback on your performance.

Passive Nonverbal Behavior

The head nurse sits behind her desk or maintains an exaggerated distance from the employees. She is contantly examining and fumbling with a pen. She glances up occasionally but avoids making eye contact. Her facial expression is tense, with a nervous smile. Her voice is weak and the tone is apologetic. She hesitates frequently, and her statements often end with the inflection of a question, as if asking for approval. She giggles nervously.

Staff's reaction: What a pushover. No need to take her too seriously. Can't we get a real leader? She's going to give us feedback? Ha-ha!

Aggressive Nonverbal Behavior

The head nurse paces, walking up close to staff members with her hands on hips or pointing at individuals. Her eye contact is steady and focused for a time on each individual. Her facial expression is tense with an infrequent, forced smile. Her posture is rigid, and her voice is commanding. She speaks slowly with a tense jaw, pausing for effect and emphasizing each word.

Staff's reaction: Who does she think she is? Does she think this is the military? I don't think I'm going to like her or her feedback.

Assertive Nonverbal Behavior

The head nurse maintains a comfortable distance from the staff. Her desk is positioned so as not to present a barrier. Her hands are relaxed, either in her pockets or used for emphasis. Her eye contact is direct, moving from person to person. Her facial expression is relaxed and animated with a friendly smile. She maintains good posture and appears comfortable. Her voice is appropriately loud. She speaks clearly with a confident tone.

***Staff reaction*: This sounds interesting. I'd better pay attention. She sounds like she means business. Maybe we can get something done around here now. I think she is someone I can respect.**

It is important to point out that no single behavior makes a message passive, aggressive, or assertive. It is the total effect that is significant. You also need to identify the original intent or goal of the communication and determine if the behavior supports or nullifies that goal.

As an assertive nurse manager, you want to have the respect of your employees. You want them to take you seriously when you pass on information to them, and you do not want your nonverbal behavior to distract from or cancel out your verbal message. You want to project an image of self-assurance. Even at times when you are less than self-assured, you can, through developing these assertive verbal and nonverbal skills, appear more confident than you feel. The more confident you act, the more confident you feel, and the more confident you feel, the more confident you act.

Professional Image

Your appearance is an element of nonverbal behavior that makes a strong statement about you to others and can be either an asset or a detriment in defining your role as a manager. You can reinforce your position as a manager through the way you dress. The lab coat is the status symbol of the health care professional. For men and women, a lab coat worn over a uniform or street clothes communicates authority. If you wear a uniform, choose the most business-like style possible. Be sure that your hair, shoes, and accessories also project a professional image consistent with your responsibility as a manager.

It is impossible to avoid creating an image through your dress and nonverbal behavior. You can choose to plan an image that will enhance your role, or you can choose to ignore the image issue. Choosing to ignore the issue may result in your having to work harder to overcome an image inconsistent with your managerial responsibilities.

4

Managerial Listening Response
Two ears and one mouth

"The Lord gave us two ears and one mouth.
I guess that means He wants us to do about
twice as much listening as talking."

To listen more is good advice. However, as a busy nurse manager you must be concerned about using your listening time efficiently and effectively to benefit you, your employees, and your organization. You are already familiar with these assertive nonverbal listening behaviors:

- Use of frequent eye contact, while avoiding an anxiety–producing stare
- Adoption of a relaxed, receptive body posture
- Elimination of barriers such as a desk between you and the speaker

Listening Styles

In order to be an effective listener, you must also *respond* to what you are hearing. Just as the style of your verbal and nonverbal communication can be identified as passive (no conflict), aggressive (get what I want), or assertive (communication without violation), your managerial listening response can also be categorized according to these styles.

Following is an illustration of an employee with a personal problem and three different styles of listening response by the nurse manager. Which response will, in the long run, be most beneficial to both the employee and the organization?

Situation

A staff nurse approaches the head nurse in the nurse's station.

Staff Nurse: **Ms. Scott, I've got lots of problems at home. You know my husband left me and now that teenage son of mine wants to stay out all hours. I'm not sleeping well, and I feel so tired all the time I can barely drag myself to work. Yesterday I started crying when I was giving Mr. Richards his bath.**

Listening Response: Passive (no conflict)

Head Nurse: **Oh, Mrs. Williams, I'm so sorry. You know I'm always concerned about my staff. It was thoughtless of me to give you a heavy assignment. I understand how**

**upsetting these family problems can be. I should be more
supportive. Let's go in my office right now and talk about
it. You probably need to get some things off your chest.**

**Don't be concerned about your assignment. I'll ask
someone else to cover for you. We'll talk as long as you
need to. Now don't you worry because everything will
work out just fine.**

The nurse manager using this style of listening
response is likely to spend more actual time listening than
either of the other two. Quantity, however, does not necessarily equal quality. Since her goal is no conflict, her listening is hampered by her heightened anxiety. Instead of
focusing on the needs of the employee, she is focused on
herself. She is more concerned about saying the right thing
than listening for the right thing. She places unrealistic
demands upon herself: "I should know the answer to all
things." In an effort to be well liked, she has difficulty setting time or topic limitations with her employees. She
generally offers reassurance rather than exploring new
ideas. Reassurance is safe and easy and makes the
employee feel better for the moment.

Listening Response: Aggressive
(get what I want)

Head Nurse: **(talking while still writing in chart) Oh,
I'm sorry to hear that. I'll tell you what I did when my
husband left. I said, "Good riddance!" As for that
teenager, I'd just remind him who is paying the bills. Tell
you what, we've got a lot of work to do around here, but I
can assign Mr. Richards to one of the other nurses since
you're having so much trouble with men these days.**

HAROLD BRIDGES LIBRARY
S. MARTIN'S COLLEGE
LANCASTER

This highly task-oriented and organization-conscious nurse manager views talking as a waste of time, unless she is doing most of it. In order to meet her goal of getting what she wants, she is often too hurried and preoccupied to listen carefully. Like the passive nurse manager, she is focused on her own needs. Unlike the passive manager who is thinking "I should," however, the aggressive manager is thinking "I want—she should." After only half-listening, she decides what her employee's goals should be and even how she should feel. Frequently she will cut off an employee's expression of concern with a quickly formulated answer or rebuttal. She tends to minimize employee's problems and feelings. Her responses are often characterized by detailed personal examples and unsolicited advice.

Listening Response: Assertive (communication without violation)

Head Nurse: **(puts down chart and gives employee full attention) It certainly sounds like you're going through some hard times right now. I'm glad you told me and I think we need to talk more. Let's meet in my office for about a half-hour right after you get back from lunch today. I'll get Ms. Ellis to watch your patients for you during that time. I think I can suggest some resources that may be very useful to you.**

The time spent in listening by the assertive nurse manager is influenced by her attempts to maintain a balance between a concern for her employees and the needs of the organization. Whenever possible she structures specific times for listening so that she can give the employee her full attention without interfering with the performance of duties.

HAROLD RINGLE LIBRARY
S. MARTIN'S COLLEGE
LANCASTER

Her self-confidence allows her to focus on the speaker and to actively process the information as she listens. She asks appropriate questions, both to obtain information and to help the employee solve problems. She realizes that employees must arrive at their own goals and solutions. She may choose to offer restrained, well-thought-out personal experiences that can be reassuring or serve as models of behavior.

The assertive nurse manager remains consistent in her role as a manager and avoids slipping into a counselor role. Any feedback given to employees is related to job performance. If the employee is experiencing personal problems, the assertive nurse manager assesses for the possible existence of a crisis situation. She then proceeds to make appropriate referrals to assist the employee in the resolution of the problem.

Like other assertive skills, the assertive managerial listening response can be perfected through practice. With your peers, you may wish to practice role-playing appropriate listening responses to common managerial situations.

5

Rational Thinking
*Management can be fun—
I think*

Yes, management can be fun—if you learn to control your thinking. "Men are disturbed not by things, but the view they take of them" (Epictetus, 1st century A.D.). "Nothing is either good or bad but thinking makes it so" (William Shakespeare). No one has the power to upset us. You can control your emotional responses to any situation by controlling your thoughts about the situation. Albert Ellis, the pioneer of rational thinking, describes the ABC's of emotions as:

A. Situation or event (what happened)
B. Self-talk, thoughts, attitudes, and beliefs (interpretation of what happened)
C. Consequences (feelings and actions).

Using the ABC's to Improve Employee Relations

A. *Situation*

You are a new head nurse and one of your R.N.'s has come in 20 minutes late for the past three mornings. You talk with her and she says it won't happen again. The very next morning she is 20 minutes late.

B. *Your self-talk, thoughts, beliefs about the situation*

I can't believe she's late again. Doesn't she think I mean business? I told her she had to be on time. She's doing this on purpose because I'm new. She thinks I won't do anything. She thinks she can get by with this. I'll show her. She can't treat me this way.

C. *Consequences*

You feel very angry and defensive. You yell at the R.N. in the presence of other staff members. You inform her that you will not tolerate this behavior and that you're going to write her up.

It is very clear in this example that the head nurse's thoughts and beliefs about the situation resulted in irrational anger and inappropriate behavior. Ellis suggests learning to challenge your thoughts. Ask yourself questions about your thoughts and determine if they are rational or irrational. Irrational thinking is based on emotions. Rational thinking is based on objective reality. Rational thinking helps you to reach your goals and decreases conflict with others. The head nurse in the example could challenge her irrational thoughts in the following way:

Irrational Thought: Doesn't she think I mean business? I told her to be on time.

Challenge: I need to find out what the problem is since we did discuss her tardiness yesterday.

Irrational Thought: She's doing this on purpose because I'm new.

Challenge: I don't know that for sure. She's been pleasant and helpful to me in other situations.

Irrational Thought: She thinks I won't do anything. She thinks she can get by with this. I'll show her.

Challenge: I need to talk with her and make sure she understands the consequences if she continues to be late.

Irrational Thought: She can't treat me this way.

Challenge: I have no evidence that she is trying to "do anything to me." The only facts I have are that she was 20 minutes late.

Consequences Resulting from Challenging Irrational Thoughts: Although you are angry, you are not irrational. You calmly tell the R.N. that you want to talk with her in private after report. When you meet with her you evaluate the facts, let her know how you feel about her behavior and let her know the consequences if this behavior continues.

If you learn to challenge and control your thoughts then you can control your emotional reaction to conflict situations. If you are in control of your feelings, then you can choose a more rational, assertive response. Remember, facts don't cause feelings. It's your thoughts and beliefs about situations that cause feelings, and feelings lead to actions.

Ellis suggests the camera-check technique to help you learn to evaluate situations accurately. A camera shows a situation the way it is. It reveals the facts without making interpretations or judgments. Your response to employees should be based on facts, not on your thoughts or beliefs about the facts. If you base your response on facts, you can take more appropriate assertive action with your employees.

Positive Imaging

You can use positive imaging to assist you in decreasing your anxiety and planning strategies. If you think of yourself as a surfer and your management problems as waves, you will learn to welcome the challenges. Surfers cannot possibly ride every wave. They have to watch the swells carefully to know if and when to make their moves. They have to anticipate the size of the wave and decide whether to ride it or let it pass by.

Surfers don't attempt to ride every small wave, and a nurse manager knows that many problems are best handled by benign neglect. Accomplished surfers watch the calm seas in anticipation of a swell. They make preparation to catch the wave early and ride it to its crest. Just as the surfer watches the swells and selects the big waves, the nurse manager selects those problems that deserve her attention.

As a nurse manager you may choose to become uninvolved in minor conflicts among your staff. On the other hand you may choose to intervene quickly in conflicts that have the potential to escalate into major management problems. You need to stay on top of problems and ride them out rather than allow them to wipe you out. You will no doubt have your share of wipeouts, but you will more often experience the perfect ride when you're in control and you achieve the desired results.

It is also important for managers to learn to accentuate the positive. Positive thoughts lead to positive feelings. Instead of looking at your inevitable management or employee problems as some sort of torture that must be endured as a part of your job, try looking at these problems as expected challenges and opportunities for growth. These challenges are the reason you have a job. They are your opportunity to excel and to exercise your creativity and innovative abilities.

Climate Control

As the manager on your unit you are in charge of climate control. Rather than being a thermometer that merely reflects the prevailing climate, you can choose to be a thermostat and exert some control over the climate. Your attitude is to a large extent reflected by your staff. Your behavior as a manager will influence the behavior of your staff. You serve as a role model, so model the behavior you expect from your staff. You need to have a positive visual image of the performance you expect from yourself as a manager as well as the performance you expect from your employees. Engage in positive self-talk regarding this performance. For example, think, "Using my assertive communication skills, I expect that I will be able to assist each member of my staff in setting goals and becoming a more motivated, productive employee."

Rational thinking, positive imaging, and positive self-talk will not guarantee that your employees will always meet your expectations. Utilizing these skills, however, will increase the probability of desired performance and management will be more fun.

6

Stress Management
Curing the super-nurse syndrome

N urses who have aspired to be nurse managers are high achievers. They expect a lot of themselves, and their high expectations can lead to the super-nurse syndrome.

There is nothing wrong with working hard and doing a good job. Achievement builds our confidence and motivates us to continue our accomplishments. High achievers are usually rewarded for their hard work by approval and praise from others and by awards and promotions.

Super-nurses, however, try to accomplish more than is reasonably possible in a given time. They are perfectionists and are so identified with their work that they feel best about themselves when they are working hard. They have a hard time relaxing and enjoying the little pleasures of life. Do you have symptoms of the super-nurse syndrome?

Super-Nurse Symptoms Checklist

- ❏ Do you do everything in a hurry?
- ❏ Do you become impatient with others because they aren't working at your speed?
- ❏ Do you do more than one thing at a time? Do you read while eating, for instance, or think about work while exercising?
- ❏ Do you feel guilty when relaxing or playing?
- ❏ Do you feel that everything you do must be perfect?
- ❏ Do you believe that your worth is directly related to how much you accomplish?
- ❏ Do you overschedule your time?
- ❏ Do you get irritated when you have to wait in line or you get caught in traffic?
- ❏ Do you frequently feel too rushed to chat with a friend or enjoy a beautiful sunset?
- ❏ Do people often tell you that you need to slow down and relax?
- ❏ Do you find it difficult to ask for help or do you turn down help when it is offered?
- ❏ Do you often put off starting a task because you won't have time to do it right or finish it?

A positive response to any of these questions indicates expectations of yourself that you may wish to change. As a nurse manager it is also important for you to be aware that these high self-expectations affect how you respond to others. You have a certain tolerance for mistakes (yours and others). If you think of your tolerance for mistakes as being on a continuum it would look like this:

Apathetic Nurse Manager	Rational Nurse Manager	Super-Nurse Manager
←		→
High tolerance for mistakes	Realistic tolerance for mistakes	Low tolerance for mistakes

The apathetic nurse manager has a high tolerance for mistakes and she has a "just do enough to get by" attitude. The super-nurse manager has a low tolerance for mistakes and a "must get everything done perfectly now" attitude. While the rational nurse manager works hard to prevent any errors, she recognizes that some mistakes are inevitable and she has a "let's do the best job we can" attitude.

If you are an on-fire super-nurse manager you may find someday that you've burned out and become an apathetic nurse manager. On the other hand, you may find that you have become addicted.

Characteristics of Work Addiction

❑ Work relieves emotional and physical discomfort.
❑ There is an experience of pleasure, a "rush," which can be brought about only by work.
❑ Work becomes the center of life, and all other activities and relationships are adjusted to accommodate

it. Nothing is allowed to interfere with the pursuit of the addictive behavior.

❏ The addict believes that she needs only herself and her work to be self-sufficient.

❏ There is denial of any problems. The addict can't see what everyone else can see.

❏ If work is eliminated, there is a physical and emotional period of withdrawal, characterized by anxiety and depression, which can be relieved only by work.

When work becomes all-consuming to the point that it meets these criteria, it is called workaholism. Since abstinence is not an option for most of us, the best advice is to treat the condition in its early stages. For many nurses the super-nurse syndrome can be the onset of workaholism. How do you treat the super-nurse syndrome?

Challenging Irrational Beliefs

First, recognize that you hold some irrational beliefs about yourself and your capabilities. Some of the messages you give yourself that cause the super-nurse syndrome are:

1. I must always be perfectly competent.
2. I must work hard all the time if I'm going to be a worthwhile person.
3. I must always get things done on time.
4. I should not make mistakes.
5. People should do things the right way (my way).

Next, challenge these negative irrational thoughts and substitute positive rational thoughts. The irrational components in all of the statements above are the words *should*, *must*, and *always*. These words generate guilt and anxiety. Eliminate them from your vocabulary, and use words such as *want*, *choose*, and *prefer*. For example, if you find yourself feeling like you must always be perfectly competent, remind yourself that it is impossible to do everything perfectly always. There are times you won't know the answer to a question or you'll make a mistake. No one is perfect. We all make mistakes. Believing you must be perfect creates anxiety within you, which increases the probability of mistakes and inhibits you from taking risks. It also leads to procrastination, because you keep putting tasks off until you have time to do them perfectly. Challenging your irrational thoughts in this manner is a stress management skill that you can develop with practice.

Essential Rules of Time Management

Much of your job stress is probably related to trying to fulfill your responsibilities and meet your deadlines. Since we all have exactly the same amount of time and there is nothing we can do to stretch it, the challenge becomes one of *managing* time. If you don't control your time, your time will control you, resulting in more stress. There are two essential rules of time management: prioritize and delegate.

Accept the fact that as a nurse manager you will never have time to do all the things you want to do. Therefore, it is extremely important for you to set priorities. Turla and Hawkins (1982) suggest that you make elephant hunting your highest priority and minimize ant stomping. In other words, you go after the big, high-payoff goals and minimize the time you spend on little, low-payoff goals. Start every day by making a to-do list and deciding what your elephants (E) and ants (A) are and what can be delegated (D) to someone else. Simply mark the items on your list E, A, or D.

It's important to recognize that in order to get the job done you need help. Use D's liberally. Remember you can't do everything. Make sure you spend most of your time on elephants. Delegate as many of the ants as possible. Don't feel guilty about the use of delegation; it is a very useful staff development tool. By utilizing the skill of delegation you can assign tasks to others that build on their strengths and further their professional growth. Taking into consideration your staff's individual professional goals will make your delegation even more effective. So delegation is not a way of getting out of work, it's a way to help your staff.

After you have determined what your elephants are, remember that the way to eat an elephant is one bite at a time. In other words, make use of small blocks of time to get started. Don't wait until you have time to eat the entire elephant. You will find yourself pleasantly surprised at how much progress you can make if you utilize those small blocks of time.

You will need to frequently reassess your to-do list, crossing out tasks completed, adding items, and reassigning priorities. An ant on today's list may become an elephant tomorrow. For example, you may receive some communication from your supervisor that changes the priority of an item, or an incident may occur on your ward that necessitates making an item higher priority.

Conclusion

Giving yourself positive rational messages, prioritizing, and delegating are the secrets of stress management that will help you cure the super-nurse syndrome. Reducing your own stress will make you a more effective nurse manager.

7

Motivation
Creating a team

One of the most exciting and rewarding functions of a nurse manager is that of motivating employees. "But trying to motivate employees is my greatest frustration," you may argue. Perhaps we can help. "Motivate" means to provide with a motive and "motive" comes from the root word motion which is an incentive to act. People are motivated when they are provided with incentives they can internalize as their own. Discovering these incentives in yourself and others is the key to motivation.

Recipe for Motivation

Salary is the most obvious incentive. A familiar bumper sticker says it all: "I owe, I owe, so off to work I go!" But salary alone does not make work interesting or exciting. A Recipe for Motivation includes the following steps:

Step I.   Start with a vision and shape it into a goal.
Step II. Blend with a larger cause or group effort.
Step III. Serve with a feeling of accomplishment.
Step IV. Garnish with appreciation and recognition.

Motivating Yourself

The main difference between leaders and followers is the leaders' ability to have a vision of the future, to set goals, and to keep themselves excited about these goals. In other words, as a manager you must first motivate yourself. The following illustrates how utilizing the Recipe for Motivation can keep one nurse manager a "Motivated Molly," while failure to use the recipe results in another nurse manager's becoming a "Burned-Out Betsy."

Motivated Molly

Step I. **Molly has a written list of long-range and short-term goals for herself, her staff, and her unit. Many of these goals have been generated from discussion with her staff. Molly's goals were developed from the following areas of interest.**

    A. Personal

        1. Increase research activity in order to meet promotion criteria

        2. Increase family ties

        3. Keep work current (employee performance evaluations, for example)

    B. Staff

        1. Assist staff in becoming certified

        2. Increase staff responsibility

         3. Develop leadership skills in the staff

     C. Unit

         1. Provide adequate staffing on each shift

         2. Decrease absenteeism

         3. Develop a collaborative, collegial relationship between physicians and nurses

Step II. Molly is involved in working with other nurse managers at her facility to provide a stimulating work environment for nurses as part of the hospital's recruitment and retention program. She is also part of a state nurses' association workgroup to promote professionalism in nursing.

Step III. Because Molly has written goals she is able to clearly identify her accomplishments. Her self-esteem and self-confidence are heightened.

Step IV. She receives recognition for her work because she is assertive in crediting herself for her accomplishments.

Burned-Out Betsy

Step I. Betsy probably has some goals in mind for herself, her staff, and her unit, but they are not clearly formulated or written down. Her goal each day is to get the work done without a crisis. She is too disorganized to think in long-range terms and to involve her staff in goal setting.

Step II. She is too busy getting the day's work done to attend nurse manager meetings or get involved in hospital and professional committees that affect nursing.

Step III. Without written goals, Betsy is unable to identify her accomplishments.

Step IV. **Betsy works hard putting out fires every day and does little to distinguish herself. Therefore, she seldom receives recognition and frequently feels unappreciated.**

New nurse managers assume their roles with excitement about possibilities for the future. However, their enthusiasm can quickly be stolen by the everyday stress of being a manager. Two thieves of motivation are (1) discouragement from unrealistic expectations of self and others and (2) stress due to poor time management. You can defend yourself from these thieves by carefully selecting the problems you address and by practicing the skills of rational thinking, prioritizing, and delegating. Of course, keeping a positive outlook goes hand in hand with keeping yourself motivated. As manager/motivator, you inspire people to put forth their best efforts by first putting forth your best efforts.

The following is a situation that any nurse manager could face. As the example illustrates, however, having a recipe for motivation allows you to handle a stressful day in a way that is not demotivating.

Situation

The nurse manager reports for duty and finds a note from the night shift stating that the coffee pot burned out. Two staff nurses call in sick, and two staff nurses are arguing. One threatens to go home if she has to work with "that nurse." Dr. Jane Smith interrupts the morning nursing report and asks to speak to the nurse manager about a patient. The nurse manager receives a call from the nursing office reminding her that five performance evaluations are due tomorrow. Checking

her appointments for the day the nurse manager realizes that she has a lunch meeting with a staff nurse to discuss the nurse's goal to become certified. She has plans to go out to dinner with her husband.

Burned-out Betsy Reacts: "This is awful. I won't be able to handle all of this. This shouldn't be happening to me. It's not fair." She begins by checking out the coffee pot. She decides it cannot be repaired and makes plans to utilize her lunch time to purchase a new one. She cancels her lunch meeting with the staff nurse, telling the nurse that she will reschedule at a later date. She looks at her limited staffing schedule for the day and decides that she will have to be the medication nurse. During report she tells the two staff nurses who have been arguing that she does not have time to listen to their dispute and she expects them to get on with their work. Anticipating a problem, she responds to the doctor's interruption by leaving report and spends 15 minutes talking to her about the patient. She has two performance evaluations completed that she worked on at home last night. She was going to complete the other three at work today, but decides she will have to take them home and do them tonight. She calls her husband and cancels their dinner plans.

Motivated Molly Responds: This nurse manager takes a few minutes alone in her office to review her priority list, which she made out the night before, and to check her calendar. She responds by thinking: "There's a lot going on here this morning. I can best handle it by being realistic about what I can accomplish, setting priorities, and delegating." Before going to report she notifies her supervisor that two of her staff nurses called in sick. The supervisor sends her one L.P.N. as a relief. She decides

to let the L.P.N. give medications and she assigns the two staff nurses who are arguing to opposite sides of the ward. She asks each of them to come to her office at 10:00 A.M. in an attempt to identify and resolve their disagreement. When the doctor interrupts the report, she explains that she will have the R.N. assigned to the patient meet with the doctor after report. She has been working on performance evaluations at work every day and has completed all but one. She has set completion of this one as a high priority today. She keeps the lunch appointment with the staff nurse to discuss her goal to be certified. She asks one of the staff nurses to have the coffee pot checked out and let her know what needs to be done. She leaves a message for the night shift that the problem is being resolved. She spends one hour working on her research project regarding empathy. Before leaving work she checks completed tasks off her to-do list and makes a new list for tomorrow. She calls her husband to confirm their dinner plans.

These examples illustrate how two nurse managers deal with the same set of circumstances. The difference in their responses is that Molly follows the Recipe for Motivation. Both nurses, Molly and Betsy, began their careers with a desire to succeed. Molly has been able to channel her energy so that she can move progressively toward the achievement of her goals. Through her guidance and role modeling she is now able to successfully motivate her employees.

If you are already experiencing symptoms of burnout, you may wonder how you can remotivate yourself. The Recipe for Motivation is still the answer. As you begin to set goals you may be lacking in enthusiasm. However, feelings follow actions. The act of setting goals will start you on your way to feeling more motivated. If you are having problems even thinking of goals, use your staff as resources. Brainstorming with them will not only generate goals but will also be stimulating and motivating for everyone involved.

Motivating Employees

Within all employees there is a potential spark of excitement about their jobs. The nurse manager with a highly motivated staff has provided the proper environment for the spark to ignite into flames. Most employees want an opportunity to benefit the organization they work for and to reach their own full potential. The successful manager/motivator is creative in providing these opportunities for her employees. She utilizes the Recipe for Motivation.

> *Step I.* **She helps her staff identify their own goals and encourages them to adopt challenging new goals for themselves and the organization. She works with them individually and in groups to formulate these goals in writing.**
>
> *Step II.* **She clearly communicates to her staff her goals for the unit. She informs them of the organization's goals and interprets for them the part they play in the achievement of their goals.**
>
> *Step III.* **By reviewing goals and giving feedback, she is able to help her staff identify progress, and she enhances their sense of accomplishment, thereby increasing their self-esteem and self-confidence.**
>
> *Step IV.* **She gives appreciation and recognition whenever it is appropriate. She is careful to be conservative in her praise so that it will not lose its**

effectiveness. She also expects employees to write self-evaluations and to give themselves credit for their achievements.

The following are examples of what employees can accomplish when a manager/motivator helps them identify goals and provides the proper environment and opportunity for the goals to be accomplished.

1. **The nurse manager on Ward 8 North encouraged her staff to set a goal to win the hospital's poster contest for Nursing Recognition Week. All staff members submitted ideas for a theme and she designated a committee to design the finished product. The committee agreed to work on the poster off duty, while the nurse manager agreed to schedule one hour compensatory time for each member. The prize was a pizza party for all shifts, as well as having their poster on display in the hospital lobby.**
2. **When staff in a critical-care unit expressed concern about the resignation of two staff nurses who had been on the unit less than six months, the nurse manager encouraged them to take some action. They set a goal to develop a plan that would help them better meet the needs of new employees. All staff were included in generating ideas, developing the plan, and implementing it when a new employee was hired for their area. At the end of one year, all vacancies were filled, and there had been no resignations of new employees.**
3. **The nurse manager at an adolescent chemical-dependence rehabilitation center formulated a goal that nursing staff would be encouraged to become more involved in community education. She shared this goal with her staff and they put together a program, which included a skit and brief lecture aimed at helping parents teach their children to avoid drugs and alcohol. The nurses contacted**

local schools, parents' groups, and other community organizations to offer prevention programs free of charge. They experienced a great deal of satisfaction from the appreciation expressed to them by those attending the programs. At the end of the year, the nurse manager recommended to the center director that each nurse who participated receive a cash bonus.

Having no purpose or direction results in boredom and lethargy. Having clearly defined goals results in energy and action. As a nurse manager interested in increasing your employee motivation, you need to set goals with your employees, give them feedback, and use the power of your position to create challenging opportunities and supportive networks in which they can participate. Through your efforts, not only can your employees meet the needs for which they were hired, they can also grow professionally and develop to their full potential.

Conclusion

As a manager/motivator you are working to keep yourself motivated and you are also working *for* your staff to provide them with incentives for action. Through your efforts you and your staff will become a TEAM.

*T*errifically

*E*nergized

*A*nd

*M*otivated!

8

Goal Setting

If you don't know where you are going, how will you know when you get there?

If you have achieved the level of nurse manager, you are already a goal setting and goal achieving individual. Since you first conceived the idea of becoming a nurse, you have set and achieved a large number of personal goals. Now, as a nurse manager, your success and satisfaction are in direct proportion to your ability to set goals for your unit and to assist your staff in setting individual, work related goals.

As the chapter title implies, a journey without a destination would result in weary, frustrated travelers. Likewise, a nursing unit without clearly formulated goals will result in weary, frustrated and eventually burned-out staff members who rush through a work day without direction. They will miss the satisfaction of arrival that comes when a goal has been achieved. They will spend time and expend energy but will define little progress or few accomplishments other than making it through the day. Goal setting allows people to experience success. People don't plan to fail—they just fail to plan.

Goal Setting Categories

Your goal setting activities, as a nurse manager, will fall into three categories.

1. Organization Goals

The organization prescribes goals (policies) for which you must develop plans that you and your employees will follow. Sometimes even the plans are defined by the organization and handed down to you to implement (procedures).

2. Unit Goals

You will establish goals for your unit that are based on its particular needs and the interests of your employees. This can be an exciting process when all staff members participate in determining the goals and developing the plans. The journey toward the destination becomes a team effort.

3. Individual Goals

**You and your staff members have individual goals for
your own professional growth. As a nurse manager, you
act as advisor to your staff members and help them plan
a course of action involving work experience, educational
experiences, and career development opportunities.**

Goal Setting Steps

Many people fail to achieve goals because they never
get beyond the stage of wishing. A goal is a wish with a
plan of action and a deadline. As a nurse you are familiar
with the nursing process, which is a framework for goal setting. This same process can be used for setting organizational, unit, and individual goals.

Assessment

1. **Determine a destination (desired outcome).**

2. **Put the goal and action plan in writing (goal setting
   worksheet).**

Plan

3. **Map out a route or action plan for getting there (steps
   leading toward achievement).**

Intervention

4. **Put the action plan into a time frame (overall and intermediate deadlines).**

5. **Designate accountability (person or group responsible).**

Evaluate

6. **Keep current and on schedule (periodic review and revision).**

If any one of these steps is missing, the goal setting process is incomplete.

Following is a goal setting worksheet that applies these steps. We encourage you to reproduce this worksheet and put it to use on your unit. Because the goals will be written and kept current, they become the basis of feedback and progress checks with your employees. They will simplify the writing of employee evaluations and periodic unit reports. We have also given you examples of how the worksheet can be used by you and your staff to set goals.

Goal Setting Worksheet

Date

Desired Outcome

Deadline for Achievement

Steps toward Achievement	*Intermediate Deadlines*	*Name of Person or Group Responsible*

Date for Review, Revision, or Update	*Name of Person or Group Responsible*

Example #1: Organization Goal (Policy)

Goal Setting Worksheet

Date Today

Desired Outcome: An initial nursing-care plan, using approved care-plan format, will be completed on every (100%) new patient within eight hours of admission to this unit.

Deadline for Achievement* (one month from this date)

Steps toward Achievement	*Intermediate Deadlines*	*Name of Person or Group Responsible*
1. Review policy with staff on each shift at change of shift	(One week from today)	Melissa Hall, Head Nurse
2. Meet with one team leader from each shift to plan 15-minute inservice on care plans	(One week from today)	Melissa Hall, Head Nurse
3. Provide staff with up-to-date article from a nursing journal on developing care plans	(Two weeks from today)	Melissa Hall, Head Nurse
4. Provide staff with a sample care plan, which has been reviewed and approved by head nurse.	(Three weeks from today)	Miriam Bell, Staff Nurse
5. Conduct 15-minute inservice on each shift regarding care plans	(Three weeks from today)	Miriam Bell, Staff Nurse; Janice Clack, Staff Nurse; Sue Covey, Staff Nurse
6. Audit each patient record on unit for completed care plan	(Four weeks from today)	Melissa Hall, Head Nurse

*Deadlines should be as specific as possible. Use actual dates.

Date for Review, Revision, or Update	*Name of Person or Group Responsible*
(One month from today)	Melissa Hall, Head Nurse

Example #2: Unit Goal

Goal Setting Worksheet

Date Today

Desired Outcome: Ward 7 East will utilize all available space to maximum advantage in order to provide a safe, efficient, comfortable, and pleasant environment for both patients and staff.

*Deadline for Achievement** (one year from today)

Steps toward Achievement	Intermediate Deadlines	Name of Person or Group Responsible
1. Brainstorming session— each shift will be utilized to stimulate interest and to generate lists of ideas and suggestions.	(Two weeks from today)	Melissa Hall, Head Nurse, and charge nurse on each shift: Jane Brown, Sara Giles, Hope Jones
2. Assign all staff to one of the following work groups: a. patient rooms, other patient-care areas, and visitors' lounge b. staff work and break areas c. storage areas and office space	(Three weeks from today)	Melissa Hall, Head Nurse
3. Consider staff preference in assigning work group when possible. Have representation from each shift on each group. Appoint a group leader.	(Same)	Melissa Hall, Head Nurse

*Deadlines should be as specific as possible. Use actual dates.

Steps toward Achievement	*Intermediate Deadlines*	*Name of Person or Group Responsible*

4. Each work group will thoroughly explore needs and possibilities in its area by using methods such as:
  a. discuss brainstorming suggestions
  b. survey other wards and examine differences in space utilization
  c. identify and utilize resources inside the hospital (engineering, supply, building management) and outside the hospital (for example, a school of design that might need a student project)
	(Three months from today)	group leaders

5. Work group leaders present head nurse with list of identified needs and projected solutions. Make list available for examination by all unit staff and appropriate hospital administration.	(Four months from today)	group leaders and Melissa Hall, Head Nurse

Steps toward Achievement	Intermediate Deadlines	Name of Person or Group Responsible
6. Using Goal Setting Worksheet, each group leader will develop a plan for achievement of goals over the next seven months.	(Five months from today)	group leaders

Date for Review, Revision, or Update		Name of Person or Group Responsible
(4th Wednesday of each month until goal is achieved)		group leaders

Example #3: Individual Work-Related Goal

Goal Setting Worksheet

Date Today

Desired Outcome: Mary Smith, R.N., will be certified by the American Nurses Association (ANA) as a Clinical Specialist in Adult Medical Surgical Nursing.

Deadline for Achievement* (Date of Certification Examination)

Steps toward Achievement	*Intermediate Deadlines*	*Name of Person or Group Responsible*
1. Write ANA for application	(One week from today)	Mary Smith
2. Arrange authorized absence for date of examination	(One month from today)	Mary Smith
3. Make out a study and review schedule	(Two months from today)	Mary Smith
4. Obtain nursing endorsements, transcripts, etc.	(Two months from today)	Mary Smith
5. Study and review material according to schedule	(Date of examination)	Mary Smith
6. Successfully complete the certification examination	(Date of examination)	Mary Smith
7. Celebrate	(Weekend after examination)	Mary Smith's significant other, Edward

Date for Review, Revision, or Update		*Name of Person or Group Responsible*
As needed		Mary Smith

*Deadlines should be as specific as possible. Use actual dates.

9

Feedback
Staying on course

Most managers would agree that feedback is essential in order to keep employees on course and help them to reach their goals. However, giving employees feedback is difficult for many managers. Effective managerial feedback is *verbal and nonverbal communication with employees regarding their performance and is based on mutually agreed upon goals.*

Three Purposes of Managerial Feedback

1. To help employees know how effective they have been in achieving their performance goals.
2. To direct subsequent behavior, so that employees stay on course toward their desired goals.
3. To stimulate changes in employees' feelings, attitudes, perceptions, knowledge, and behavior.

Seven Guiding Principles

There are some basic principles to guide you as a nurse manager when you are navigating your employees toward your mutual goals. We call them the seven T's of managerial feedback: Told, Timely, Timed, Targeted, Tactful, Truthful, and Tuned.

1. Told

Managers should inform employees that they will be given feedback regarding their performance. Feedback is best received when asked for, but at the very least it should be expected. Employees should know that they will receive both scheduled performance evaluations and unscheduled, spontaneous feedback.

2. Timely

Positive behavior is more apt to be reinforced and negative behavior more likely to be corrected if feedback closely follows the behavior.

3. Timed

A manager should be sensitive to an employee's particular circumstances and readiness to hear the feedback. If, for example, you know that one of your employees has just been informed of a personal loss, that is not the time to give her negative feedback about her performance.

4. Targeted

Feedback should be specific. When feedback is given in a very general way it tends to frustrate the individual since she may not know to what specific behavior you are alluding. Try not to use judgmental words such as "good" or "bad." Give a description of the behavior in measurable and objective terms.

Avoid bringing up comments from past evaluations. Stay in the here and now. Feedback should be related to performance goals. Nurse managers should avoid making critical remarks about their employees' personalities. Managerial feedback should always be work related and aimed at behaviors over which the person has control.

5. Tactful

It is important that you make every effort to give feedback in such a way that it can be received without being a threat to your employee. If the employee feels threatened, she gets defensive and cannot hear or make use of the information you are giving. Feedback should be given in a neutral manner. Use I-messages and check your nonverbal as well as verbal behavior to make sure it is not threatening.

6. Truthful

When giving feedback, nurse managers should be open, honest, and direct regarding their feelings. Feedback should, however, be motivated primarily by a desire to

help the other person, not solely to satisfy your own need to express feelings.

7. Tuned

Feedback should be checked to ensure clear communication. Have your employee rephrase the feedback to see if she heard your intended message. Many people lack skills in receiving feedback and may distort your message.

Types of Feedback

There are two types of feedback—*positive*, which gives the message "You are right on course. Keep it up!" and *negative*, which gives the message "You're off course. Adjust." Contrary to what you might expect, most managers give negative feedback much more freely than positive feedback. They tend to ignore their employees when they are doing a good job and really let them have it when they make a mistake. They operate under the no-news-is-good-news philosophy. This approach does not help employees reach their full potential. It tends to discourage risk taking and stifles creativity. Positive feedback, on the other hand, is encouraging and stimulates people to strive to do even better.

Positive Feedback

We observed a beautiful example of positive feedback between a 3-year-old boy and his 8-month-old sister. He was very eager for his lttle sister to learn to crawl and play with him in his room. The sister was at the doorway of her brother's room one morning rocking back and forth on all fours, getting ready to crawl. Her big brother saw her and went running to her. He immediately started coaching her to crawl. From the next room we could hear him saying "You can do it, Sis. I know you can. Come on." We could hear his sister giggle with delight at the attention and encouraging words. (How do you think your employees would react if you let them know that you notice their efforts, even in the beginning stages, and believe in them and their ability to do a good job?)

We looked around the corner at them and saw the big brother get on his hands and knees and proceed to show his sister how to crawl. "See, this is the way to do it. Come on. There's lots of toys in my room. I'll let you play with them." (Wouldn't it be great if you gave your employees this kind of personal assistance and incentive when they're struggling with a difficult task?)

The sister continued rocking on all fours and finally crawled or wiggled her way into her brother's room. He was elated. We could hear him shouting, "I knew you could! You did great, Sis." And with that he gave her a big hug. Sis was smiling all over, obviously delighted with her brother's feedback.

What motivation to change a behavior! When you begin to spark that same kind of enthusiasm in your employees, just think of the things they will accomplish.

The following are fine points of positive feedback:*

1. Catch your employees doing things *right.* Remember your job as a manager is to help your employees succeed.

2. When employees are new on the job, remember to praise performance that is approximately right. This way you help to guide their performance in the right direction. The reinforcement will help to make that appropriate behavior reappear and remain constant.

3. Make sure your nonverbal as well as verbal behavior clearly communicates to your employees that you believe in them and feel good about their contributions to the organization.

Negative Feedback

Although positive feedback will help to keep your employees moving straight ahead toward mutually agreed upon goals, there will be times when employees will get off course and adjustments will need to be made. In those instances it is important to be able to give your employees negative feedback. In an effort to soften the blow, many managers use the "sandwich approach" in giving negative feedback. They call their employees in for a navigational adjustment and begin by giving them a compliment, followed by negative feedback, followed by another compliment. It might happen something like this:

---

*The fine points of positive and negative feedback are adapted from Blanchard K, Johnson S. *The One Minute Manager.* New York, Berkley Books, 1986.

Situation: The nurse manager calls the employee into her office for the purpose of correcting her poor documentation of patient teaching.

Nurse Manager: **Jane, you did a good job with Mr. Adams's dressing this morning, but you need to improve your documentation. I reviewed some of your charts last week and your documentation is not complete enough in regard to patient teaching. Oh by the way, I want you to know I really appreciate your being willing to work over this weekend.**

This feedback is too diluted to really have an impact. The manager started off with positive feedback and diluted it by immediately following it with a criticism. The criticism was also weakened by following it immediately with positive feedback. When the sandwich approach is used repeatedly, the employee learns to dread every compliment, for fear that it is merely a set-up for a criticism.

The following fine points of negative feedback suggest an alternative to the sandwich approach.

1. Be very specific in telling people what they did wrong.
2. Let them know verbally and nonverbally how you feel about what they did wrong.
3. Pause and remain silent for a few seconds in order to let your employees feel your displeasure.
4. Verbally and nonverbally let them know that you value them and are on their side.
5. Make sure they understand that you are upset with their performance in this particular situation, but that you still think well of them.

6. Once you have given your employees the negative feedback, put it aside. Don't continue dwelling on it.

In the next example, the nurse manager gives the employee the same criticism using these fine points of negative feedback.

Nurse Manager: **Jane, I reviewed your charts this weekend and I found that you need to improve your documentation of patient teaching. It is not enough to chart that you taught the patient. You must give some details about what you taught and his reaction. I was disappointed to find your charting incomplete. (Pauses and touches Jane on the arm.) Jane, I've seen you do a good job of teaching patients. I know you can also do a good job of documenting.**

Conclusion

As the nurse manager you are the captain of your ship. If you follow the general principles of giving feedback and incorporate the finepoints of positive and negative feedback, you will have mastered the art of keeping your crew on course. We wish you smooth sailing.

Part 2

Putting
It
All
Together

10

Clinical Skills Versus Management Skills

With everything else you have to do, why would you adopt a monkey?

You are now familiar with the essential skills that will make you a more effective nurse manager. You have a definition of an assertive nurse manager and through positive self-talk and imaging you can see yourself moving in that direction. But you have more than just the mental picture of yourself as an assertive nurse manager—you know the skills involved in assertive communication. You know how to set goals with your employees and how to give them the feedback that will keep them motivated toward better performance.

Your confidence as a manager will increase as you become more and more skillful in expressing yourself assertively. Your employees will be more satisfied and thus more productive, and you will gain the respect of both management and staff. You will not always get exactly what you want from others, but because you are assertive you will have the satisfaction of knowing that you have made your best effort.

The Monkey Trap

Even with all of this knowledge and skill, because you are a *nurse* manager, you are at risk. Your previous training, experience, and possibly even your personality traits, all make you particularly vulnerable to be caught in a "monkey trap."* That is the trap you fall into each time you take on a responsibility (monkey) that belongs to your employee. You have adopted your employee's monkey.

As mentioned previously, most nurse managers have training and experience in managing patients but do not have formal training in managing employees. When a nurse is put into an unfamiliar situation and asked to function, she will call upon familiar skills and apply them as best she can. Clinical skills, however, are different from management skills. It is the attempt to apply clinical skills to the management situation that can trap you unaware into the adoption of monkeys.

You cannot *nurse* your employees. As a manager you must *manage*. The nurse's primary role is to meet the needs of the patient. The manager's primary role is to meet the needs of the organization through helping employees reach their full potential. The trap for the nurse manager begins with her training and ability to empathize. Empathy is a

---

*The "monkey concept" is adapted from Oncken W. Get those monkeys off your back. *Working Woman* April, 1985, p. 116.

necessary skill in caring for patients and can certainly be helpful in relating to employees. But it can also interfere with the nurse's ability to manage. It is so easy to feel guilty when you can't solve employees' problems or when you have to ask employees to do something in spite of their problems.

Every time you do something for an employee that she can do for herself, you rescue her. When you take the "next move" that rightfully should be hers, you have adopted her monkey. With adoption goes responsibility. Now the monkey is yours to feed and care for. Interestingly, now that you have adopted her monkey, the employee becomes your supervisor—stopping by from time to time to see how well you are taking care of your (her) responsibility. You already have your own monkeys to care for (your responsibilities as a manager). If you fall into the monkey trap you may find yourself adopting many monkeys and doing a poor job of tending to your own. But even more important to realize is that by adopting the employee's monkey you are interfering with her right to benefit the organization and to reach her full potential.

Avoiding the Monkey Trap

How can you successfully avoid the monkey trap? How can you manage so that every employee knows her own monkeys (job expectations) and is responsible for their care and feeding? When an employee offers her monkey for adoption you have two alternatives, depending on the nature of the problems the employee is having. You must first determine if the employee *can do* or *can't do*.*

---

*Adapted from Blanchard K, Lorber R. *Putting the One Minute Manager to Work*. New York, William Morrow and Company, 1984, p. 33.

Can Do

If the employee knows her responsibility and has the necessary knowledge and skill to perform but for some reason is not performing, you, as her manager, should assume a supportive leadership style. You should be understanding and talk about her alternatives. You may go back to the goals you have mutually set and give her feedback regarding her performance. After talking with you, the employee leaves with a clear understanding of what is expected and has some ideas as to how to solve her problems. But above all, she takes her monkey with her. The next move is hers.

Situation

A new head nurse is in conference with a staff nurse who is several years her senior, in both age and work experience.

Head Nurse: Mary, I've noticed that you are late every morning. During the month I've been here you've consistently come in 10 to 15 minutes after report has begun.

Staff Nurse: (cheerfully) I've always come in at 7:45. You're so new, I guess you didn't know. I live far away and have to drop my granddaughter off at school. Everyone knows I do that. It's no problem. They all give me report later (starts to leave).

Head Nurse: It's possible that I do have some different expectations than your previous head nurse. It's important to me to get things started on time. I like to have time to help staff set goals for the day and discuss problem areas.

Staff Nurse: It's always been fine and I just don't see

how I can get here any earlier. If you want me to give up my break, I will.

Head Nurse: I understand that it will involve rearranging your personal schedule, but I do expect you to get here on time. When you arrive late it is disruptive and does not set a good example for others, and frankly I have felt very annoyed each time it's happened. (Pauses) Mary (touches her arm), as one of the senior employees on the unit, you are someone I count on to be a good role model for the younger nurses. Coming in late is not typical of your other excellent performance. Because of your experience, I had hoped to count on your help in making the daily assignments. It's very important to me that you be on time.

Staff Nurse: I didn't realize it was such a big deal. I guess I'll have to do something about it. Do you have any suggestions?

Head Nurse: No, I really don't, but you might check with Sue. She has a similar situation. Let's decide when you can expect to have the arrangements made.

Staff Nurse: Not tomorrow, for sure!

Head Nurse: I understand. Let's see, today is Monday. How about Friday? Would that give you enough time to make arrangements?

Staff Nurse: I guess so.

Head Nurse: So that we'll both be aware of your progress in this area, starting Friday I would like for you to make a note of your arrival time every day. Let's plan to meet briefly next Wednesday to see how you're doing.

Staff Nurse: Okay.

       *   *   *

Staff Nurse: It's Friday and here I am at 7:25!

Head Nurse: Why, you're the first one here! I want to tell you how good I feel about that. I know it has taken some effort to rearrange your schedule, and I appreciate it. The unit is really going to benefit from your input in planning each morning. Since you're here first, why don't you go ahead and pick your lunch time and decide who you'd like to go to lunch with.

Staff Nurse: Great!

Can't Do

You may determine, however, that an employee is having a "can't do" problem. She does not clearly understand her responsibilities, she has a different understanding of her responsibilities than you do, or she lacks the knowledge or skill to perform her responsibilities as expected. As the manager, you now assume a teaching/directive leadership style in which you may clarify goals and responsibilities, teach skills, and observe performance. It should be mentioned that there is an advantage to employees in being "slow learners." If they wear you down to the point that you become impatient, you may weaken and decide that it would be easier to adopt the monkey.

New Graduate Nurse: I've been assigned Ms. Lopez today. I've never done tracheotomy care. Somebody else will have to do that. Will you do it or ask someone to do it for me?

Head Nurse: It's important that you learn tracheotomy care. How can you best learn it?

New Graduate Nurse: Well, I've watched Mrs. Greene do tracheotomy care. I think if she helped me once or twice, I could do it.

Head Nurse: Good. I'll assign Mrs. Greene to help you today and observe you tomorrow. At the end of the shift

tomorrow we'll all three determine if you will need any further assistance with tracheotomy care.

New Graduate Nurse: **That sounds good.**

Conclusion

When you are nursing, you develop patient care plans that are tailor made, with patients assuming responsibility for their own care as they are able. When you are managing, you do not develop employee care plans. You develop plans that are designed to meet the organization's goals. The organization does not exist to meet the needs of employees. Employees are hired to meet the needs of the organization. Although some employees can assume more responsibility than others, there is a minimum expectation of all. An efficient, productive nursing organization is one in which all monkeys are attended to regularly and promptly by their rightful owners.

11

Networking
*What counts is not what you
know, but who you know who
knows what you need to know*

Within the formal structure of every organization there is an informal network. It is to your advantage as a nurse manager to understand networking and to be able to identify, utilize, and even create informal networks.

General Benefits of Networking

John Naisbitt in his 1982 best seller, *Megatrends*, defines networking as a process of "people talking to each other, sharing ideas, information and resources." As our society becomes more technological and our knowledge becomes broader, we are all called upon to become more specialized and to find ways of sharing and communicating our special areas of knowledge with each other. As workers in an organization become more independent in their areas of expertise, they become more dependent on co-workers who are experts in other areas.

In a network every person is important. Workers have an opportunity to make valuable contributions and to feel of value to the organization. Building good working relationships becomes of utmost importance because in the network management structure management and workers are all interdependent. Individual and organizational success depends upon the quality of the relationships. When networking works well, the organization becomes warm, friendly, and family like rather than cold and impersonal.

The organization benefits from networking. Workers who feel that they are able to make valuable contributions will be happier and more productive. Because workers are encouraged to cut through traditional chains of command and go directly to the source of needed information, work is performed more efficiently and effectively. John Naisbitt observes that networks can go beyond sharing information to the creation of knowledge: "As each person in a network takes in new information, he or she synthesizes it and comes up with other, new ideas."

We have all experienced the energy and creativity that can be generated when individuals are brought together in a think-tank or brainstorming situation. The outcome is usually a list of ideas of superior quantity and quality than all the individuals could have generated had they worked individually. Another positive outcome is the camaraderie that develops among group members as they stimulate each other's creativity.

Advantages of Networking for Nurse Managers

In your role as nurse manager you have been a member of nursing teams and interdisciplinary teams. You can readily utilize the concept of networking if you understand the value of shared knowledge and realize that there is strength in numbers. The nurse who attempts to be self-sufficient and all-knowing today is working *hard*. The nurse who works *smart* learns that the important thing is not *what* you know, but *who* you know who knows what you need to know. A successful nurse manager today will develop her networking abilities and will teach these skills to her staff.

When you utilize the networking process, you do not have to be the most knowlegeable clinician on your unit. Your goal, in fact, will be to develop several staff nurses who are more knowledgeable in certain areas than you are. Your challenge is to create a work environment where individuals of diverse skills and interests can grow in their own unique ways. At the same time you need to provide enough structure so that the collective efforts of all will benefit the organization.

Here are benefits that will result when you utilize the networking process.

1. Increases variety and depth of information available to the staff.
2. Makes information more accessible to the staff.
3. Provides each staff member with an opportunity to make a more valuable contribution to the unit.
4. Allows each staff member to pursue an individual area of interest.
5. Promotes better patient care because all staff members are kept up-to-date on new information.

6. Fosters team spirit by creating a team of nursing experts, each of whom is making a valuable contribution, while relying on each other for information and assistance.
7. Offers interested staff members an opportunity to assume more responsibility and to excel beyond the minimal expectations of their jobs.
8. Generates high energy, encourages creativity and innovation, and thus maintains a positive and exciting work environment.

The following is an example of a nurse manager's goal and plan to establish a network of nursing experts on her unit in a large hospital.

Goal Setting Worksheet

Date Today

Desired Outcome: Unit 5 North will develop a network of experts among R.N. staff. All staff members will choose and develop an area of interest which will be of benefit to them and the unit as a whole.

Deadline for Achievement* (One year from today)

Steps toward Achievement	*Intermediate Deadlines*	*Name of Person or Group Responsible*
1. Each R.N. chooses an area and submits it to the head nurse and assistant head nurse, who will discuss and negotiate possible duplications	(One month from today)	Each R.N., head nurse, assistant head nurse
2. A schedule of unit inservice programs will be developed so that each R.N. will make a 30-minute presentation of her area of interest within the coming calendar year	(One month from today)	Assistant head nurse
3. Each R.N. will be encouraged to attend a workshop or training session in her area of interest this year. Tuition assistance will be requested from Nursing Service	(One year from today)	Each R.N., assistant head nurse, director of nursing education

4. Each R.N. will provide the unit with current information (from journal articles and books) in her area of interest	(One year from today)	Each R.N.
5. Each R.N. will serve as a consultant to other staff members on the unit regarding her area of interest	Ongoing	Each R.N.
6. The assistant head nurse will be aware of each R.N.'s area of interest and will be responsible for connecting a nurse who has a need with the nurse who has the information	Ongoing	Assistant head nurse

Date for Review, Revision, or Update	*Name of Person or Group Responsible*
(One year from today)	Assistant head nurse

*Deadlines should be as specific as possible. Use actual dates.

12

Power
It all adds up

What are your feelings about the word POWER? Is it a positive, comfortable concept for you, or does the mention of the word make you uneasy? As you examine your feelings, you may discover that, like many nurse managers, you are ambivalent about power. In your *head* you know that having power is desirable, but in your *heart* you're not so sure. Your responses to the following statements will help you assess your reactions to power.

Reactions to Power

1. The desire for power is a normal, healthy emotion.   True ____ False ____

2. Power itself is neither good nor bad, but its use can be good or bad.   True ____ False ____

3. It is possible to exert power without violating the rights of others.   True ____   False ____

4. Power is not a masculine trait. True ____   False ____

5. You cannot have a good self-image if you feel powerless.   True ____   False ____

6 Being an expert at using power is more important to the nurse manager than being an expert clinician.
                    True ____   False ____

7. Nurses often underestimate their power.
                    True ____   False ____

8. Power comes from realistically evaluating and using all your personal assets and legitimate authority.
                    True ____   False ____

9. In order to be effective, the nurse manager must establish her own power base. True ____   False ____

10. Interpersonal alliances are helpful ways of acquiring power.   True ____   False ____

11. Powerful people are rational thinkers.
                    True ____   False ____

12. Feelings of helplessness lead to burnout.
                    True ____   False ____

13. Power is necessary to bring about change.
                    True ____ . False ____

14. It is more profitable to negotiate a compromise from a position of power.   True ____   False ____

15. The "goodies" (staff, equipment, money for continuing education) go to the people who are most visible.   True ____   False ____

As you took the test, it must have been obvious that the right answer to each question is "True." That was your intellectual reaction. Now read the test again, but this time try to get in touch with your emotional reaction. Do you equate power with negative behavior, such as intimidation and aggression? Can you acknowledge openly that having power is necessary for you to effectively perform your duties as a manager? Do you deny that having power is important, lest someone accuse you of being power hungry? Can you honestly admit, without guilt or embarrassment, that the enjoyment of power has been a motivating influence in your advancement toward the nurse manager position?

You know you need power and you probably even want it, but you are hesitant to acknowledge or use it. Your self-talk sounds something like this: "Maybe I could have some power but not tell anyone. Maybe I could exert just a little power—enough to help me handle a problem employee, but not enough to offend anyone. Maybe I could be powerful but disguise it so that the staff wouldn't notice. They would just keep on treating me like one of the gang."

You have a responsibility to your organization to fully understand and utilize the authority that has been delegated to you. You owe it to your staff to be comfortable in a position of power. The powerless cannot help the powerless. Your employees need a powerful leader. Set a goal now to become more comfortable with the power that is rightfully and necessarily yours as a nurse manager.

Three Components of Power

If you are uncomfortable with power, it is probably because you don't understand what it is. *Webster's New World Dictionary* defines power as "the ability to do, act, or produce . . . ; legal ability or authority . . ." Power is the combination of three components—authority, ability, and action. When a manager who has been given authority to lead also possesses the ability to lead and then takes action, she is exercising power. Being given authority is like having a driver's license—it is the legal capacity to act. Possessing ability is the same as having a car with a full tank of gas—it is the capability for action. But until someone takes action—turns on the ignition, presses the accelerator, and guides the car—no one goes anywhere. Consider the following formulas:

Authority + Ability – Action = Impotent manager

Authority + Action – Ability = Incompetent manager

Action + Ability – Authority = Illegitimate manager

The impotent manager uses a passive management style. Because her goal is no conflict, she avoids making decisions or taking decisive actions. By attempting to please employees, she relinquishes her power to her employees.

The incompetent manager lacks management skills such as goal setting, giving feedback, or managing time. She may not know how to avoid assuming responsibility for her employees. She may not know how to communicate or listen assertively. Her lack of ability in one or more of these areas results in increased stress and low job satisfaction for her and her employees.

The illegitimate manager uses an aggressive management style. Her main concern is results and this need may lead her to do things her way rather than following prescribed policies and procedures. Any progress may be sacrificed in the long run because of the problems created. Her illegitimate actions will also result in increased stress and low job satisfaction for her and her employees.

A powerful leader combines the authority to act with the ability to act and make things happen.

Authority + Ability + Action = Powerful Manager

When a manager takes legitimate effective action, the manager as well as the employees benefit. The manager experiences less stress and greater job satisfaction. Employees feel more secure and are more productive and better satisfied. Everyone wins, including the organization and the clients it serves.

Examples of Power

The following are examples of actions taken by powerful nurse managers:

1. A nurse manager negotiated with nursing administration to allow some of her employees to work a flexible time schedule that they requested.
2. A nurse manager informed a surgeon that one of her staff nurses had developed expertise in the physical and psychological care of patients undergoing mastectomies. They arranged for the staff nurse to present an inservice for the surgical residents, interns, and medical students.
3. A nurse manager, noticing the anxiety in the families of patients in the intensive care unit, arranged for two of her R.N.'s, a social worker, and the hospital chaplain to plan a program to better meet the needs of these family members.
4. When a physician criticized an R.N. for overstepping her bounds by bringing an unwed teenage mother

information on birth control, the nurse manager defended the nurse's role as a health care educator.

5. After noticing that patients referred from a particular hospital were often unprepared for a visit from one of her nurses, the nurse manager of a home health care agency arranged a meeting with the director of nursing from that hospital to discuss the problem. The result was a research project to investigate if patients who are prepared for the transition to home health care according to a defined protocol are less likely to be readmitted to the hospital.

6. When two R.N.'s requested approval to attend a conference but only one could be funded or spared from the unit, the nurse manager chose to approve attendance for the one whose written professional goals would be better met by attending.

Conclusion

Developing and exercising power for the benefit of yourself, your staff, and your patients means putting it all together. Your organization, by designating you as a manager, has given you authority. Your employer has shown confidence in your ability. By reading books such as this one and attending continuing education programs for nurse managers, you are further developing your management skills.

All that is left is action. So put it all together and become the powerful, assertive nurse manager that you envision yourself to be.

Bibliography

The following references have been very useful in designing our workshops for nurse managers and in developing the ideas for this book. We recommend them as valuable additional reading.

Blanchard K, Johnson S. *The One Minute Manager*. New York, Berkley Books, 1982, 1986.

Blanchard K, Lorber R. *Putting the One Minute Manager to Work*. New York, William Morrow and Company, 1984.

Clark C. *Assertive Skills for Nurses*. Rockville, MD, Aspen Productions, 1978.

Ellis A, Harper R. *A Guide to Rational Living*. North Hollywood, CA, Wilshire Books, 1974.

Lakein A. *How To Get Control Of Your Time and Your Life*. New York, Signet, 1973.

Lange A, Jakubowski P. *Responsible Assertive Behavior*. Champaign, IL, Research Press, 1976.

Molloy JT. *The Woman's Dress for Success Book*. New York, Warner Books, 1978.

Naisbitt J. *Megatrends*. New York, Warner Books, 1982.

Oncken W. Get those monkeys off your back. *Working Woman*, April, 1985, p. 116.

Oncken W. *Managing Management Time*. Englewood Cliffs, NJ, Prentice–Hall, 1984.

Peele S. *How Much Is Too Much?* Englewood Cliffs, NJ, Prentice–Hall, 1981.

Smith M. *When I Say No I Feel Guilty*. New York, Bantam Books, 1975.

Turla PA, Hawkins KL. Getting there: A personal guide to time management. *Success*, vol. 29, no. 11, 1982.

Index

An asterisk after a number indicates an
application example is included.

Addiction, work, 37–38
Aggressive behavior, listening response
    and, 26–28*
  management style and, 5, 6, 9*
  nonverbal, 21–22*
Agreeing with the possibility, 17*
Appearance of nurse manager, 24
Asking for more information, 17*
Assertive behavior, listening response
    and, 26*, 28–29*
  management style and, 5, 6,
    10–11*,11–12
  negotiation and, 18–19*
  nonverbal, 21, 23*
  nurse manager and, 3–4
  skill in, 11–12, 29
  verbal skills in, 14
    Smith on, 14
Assertive negotiation, 18–19*
Assertive nurse manager, defined, 3–4,
    11
Attitude, control of, 34
  positive, 33–34

Behavior. See specific types, e.g.,
    Aggressive behavior.
Behavior cues, 21
Burnout, 37, 44–46*

Challenging irrational beliefs, 31–32*,
    38–39
Clinical skills, vs. management skills,
    74–75, 79
Communication, goal of, 5–7, 23
  verbal, importance of, 13–14
Compromise, 18–19*
Conflict resolution, 16, 18–19, 33
Confrontation, dealing with, 17–18*
Confronting employees, 10–11*, 65,
    67–69*
Counseling, personal problems and,
    26–29*
  performance related issues and.
    See *Feedback*.
Criticism, dealing with, 17
    agreeing with possibility in, 17*
    asking for more information in,
17*
    owning the mistake in, 18*

Delegation, 39–40

Emotion, control of, 31–32*
Empathy, 74–75
Employee problems, 75–79*
Employee request, 15–16*, 18–19*

Employees' rights, 3–4, 11, 75
Encouragement. See *Feedback.*

Feedback, 3–4, 14–15
  Blanchard and Johnson on, 10, 67
  types of
    managerial, 62–65
    negative, 10–12*, 65, 67–69*,
      78–79
    performance related, 4, 29
    positive, 65–67*
Firm persistence, 15–16*
Followers, leaders vs., 43

Generalist, specialist vs., 81
Goal setting, categories of, 52–53
  employees and, 3
  steps of, 53–54
  worksheets on
    individual goal, 61*
    networking, 84–85*
    organization goal, 56–57*
    sample of, 55*
    unit goal, 58–59*
Guilt, nurse manager and, 75

I messages, 14–15, 64
Image, 23–24
Imaging, 33–34
Information, asking for, 17*
Irrational beliefs, challenging of, 31–
  32*, 38–39

Job satisfaction, 4, 11

Leaders, vs. followers, 43
Leadership, supportive style of, 76–
  78*
  teaching/directive style of, 78–79*
Learner, employee as, 78–79*
Listening, aggressive style of, 26–28*
  assertive style of, 25–26*, 28–29*
  passive style of, 26–27*

Management skills, vs. clinical skills,
  74–75, 79

Management styles, 7
Managerial feedback, 62–65
Manipulation, avoidance of, 15–18*
Mistakes, owning up to, 18*
  tolerance for, 37, 39
Monkey trap, 74–75
  avoidance of, 75–79*
  Oncken on, 74
Motivate, definition of, 42
Motivating employees, 76–79*. See
  also *Motivation recipe.*
Motivating yourself. See *Motivation
  recipe.*
Motivation recipe, 42–43
  application of
    in dealing with stress, 45–48*
    in motivating employees, 48–50*
    in motivating self, 43–45*

Negotiation, assertive, 18–19*
Networking, advantages of, 82–83
  application of, 84–85*
  definition of, 80
  general benefits of, 80–81
  Naisbitt on, 80
Nonverbal behavior, aggressive style
  of, 21–22*
  assertive style of, 21, 23*
  passive style of, 21–22*

Owning the mistake, 18*

Passive behavior, listening response
  and, 26–27*
  management style and, 6–8*
  nonverbal in, 21–22*
Performance appraisals. See *Feedback.*
Persistence, firm, 15–16*
Personal problems, employees with,
  26–29*
Power, application of, 90–91*
  components of, 88–90
  definition of, 88–89
  importance of, 88
  reactions to, 86–88
Prioritize, 39–40, 45–48*
Procrastination, 39

Professional image, 24

Rational thinking, 30–32*, 38–39
　Ellis on, 30–32
Recognition of performance, 65–67*

Self–talk, 31–32*, 34, 88
Specialist, vs. generalist, 81
— Staff development, 4, 40
　goal setting in, 52–54
　motivation and, 48–50*
　networking and, 82–83
　　unit goal, 84–85*
Stress, 6, 8, 9, 11
　dealing with
　　irrational beliefs, 39
　　motivation recipe, 45–48*
　　time management, 39–40
　symptoms of, 36

Super–nurse syndrome, symptoms of,
　36
　treatment of, 38–41

TEAM, 50
— Time management, 39–40
　Turla and Hawkins on, 39

Verbal communication, importance of,
　13–14

Work addiction (or workaholism), 37–
　38
Working smart, 82

JUNE BLANKENSHIP PUGH is a native of Atlanta, Georgia, where she received a bachelor of science degree in nursing from Emory University. She received a master of science degree from the University of Colorado with a major in psychiatric nursing. She is a member of Sigma Theta Tau and of the American Nurses' Association. She is ANA certified in adult psychiatric and mental health nursing.

Her work experience includes staff nursing on an acute-care psychiatric unit, teaching undergraduate and graduate nursing students, and directing in-service programs at Georgia Mental Health Institute. She was coordinator of a staff development program at the Veterans Administration Medical Center in Nashville, Tennessee, for five years and has taught seminars and workshops on communication skills, stress management, assertiveness, and all aspects of nurse manager–employee relations. Ms. Pugh is adjunct associate professor at Vanderbilt University School of Nursing. She is a certified substance-abuse counselor and was the clinical specialist in the alcohol treatment program at the Nashville VAMC for nine years. At present she is nursing resources coordinator, responsible for nurse recruitment and retention.

MARY ANN WOODWARD-SMITH is a native of Alabama. She received an associate degree in nursing from Calhoun State Technical Junior College in Decatur, Alabama. She received a bachelor of science degree with a major in personnel management from Athens State College in Athens, Alabama, and a master's degree in psychiatric and mental health nursing from Vanderbilt University, Nashville, Tennessee. She is a member of Sigma Theta Tau and the American Nurses' Association. She is ANA certified in adult psychiatric and mental health nursing.

She worked for six years as a nurse manager in a community mental health center, supervising a multidisciplinary staff, developing programs, and providing direct patient care. For the past eight years she has been employed at the Veterans Administration Medical Center in Nashville, Tennessee. She served as a clinical specialist on the mental health inpatient unit and is currently the coordinator of the mental health outpatient clinic. She has also been involved in the nursing department's staff development program and has led workshops and provided consultation on a variety of topics related to personal growth, management, and employee relations. Ms. Woodward-Smith is an adjunct associate professor at Vanderbilt University School of Nursing and provides clinical supervision for graduate and undergraduate students.

For more information about nurse manager/employee relations workshops or consultation, contact the authors by writing:

Nurse Manager
P. O. Box 121024
Nashville, Tennessee 37212-1024